More Bio-fuel --- Less Bio-waste

More Bio-fuel --- Less Bio-waste

Dietary Creatine Reduction Self-help Guide for People with Kidney Impairment

Wendy Lou Jones, MS, BA
Foreword by Cathi Martin, RD, CSR, LDN

Authors Choice Press
San Jose New York Lincoln Shanghai

More Bio-fuel --- Less Bio-waste
Dietary Creatine Reduction Self-help Guide
for People with Kidney Impairment

All Rights Reserved © 2001 by Wendy Lou Jones

No part of this book may be reproduced or transmitted in
any form or by any means, graphic, electronic, or mechanical,
including photocopying, recording, taping, or by any
information storage or retrieval system, without the
permission in writing from the publisher.

Authors Choice Press
an imprint of iUniverse, Inc.

For information address:
iUniverse, Inc.
5220 S. 16th St., Suite 200
Lincoln, NE 68512
www.iuniverse.com

The information and procedures contained in this book are based upon the research, as well as the professional and personal experience, of the author, and are intended for educational purposes only. They are not intended as a substituted for counseling with your physician or other health care providers. Neither the author nor the publisher is responsible for any adverse affects or consequences arising from the use of these procedures or suggestions made in this book. All matters pertaining to your physical health should be supervised by a health care professional.

ISBN: 0-595-20469-4

Printed in the United States of America

This book is dedicated to my mother, Maryann D Jones, without whose complete support in every aspect of my writing projects, none of this would be possible.

When you can't raise the bridge, lower the river.

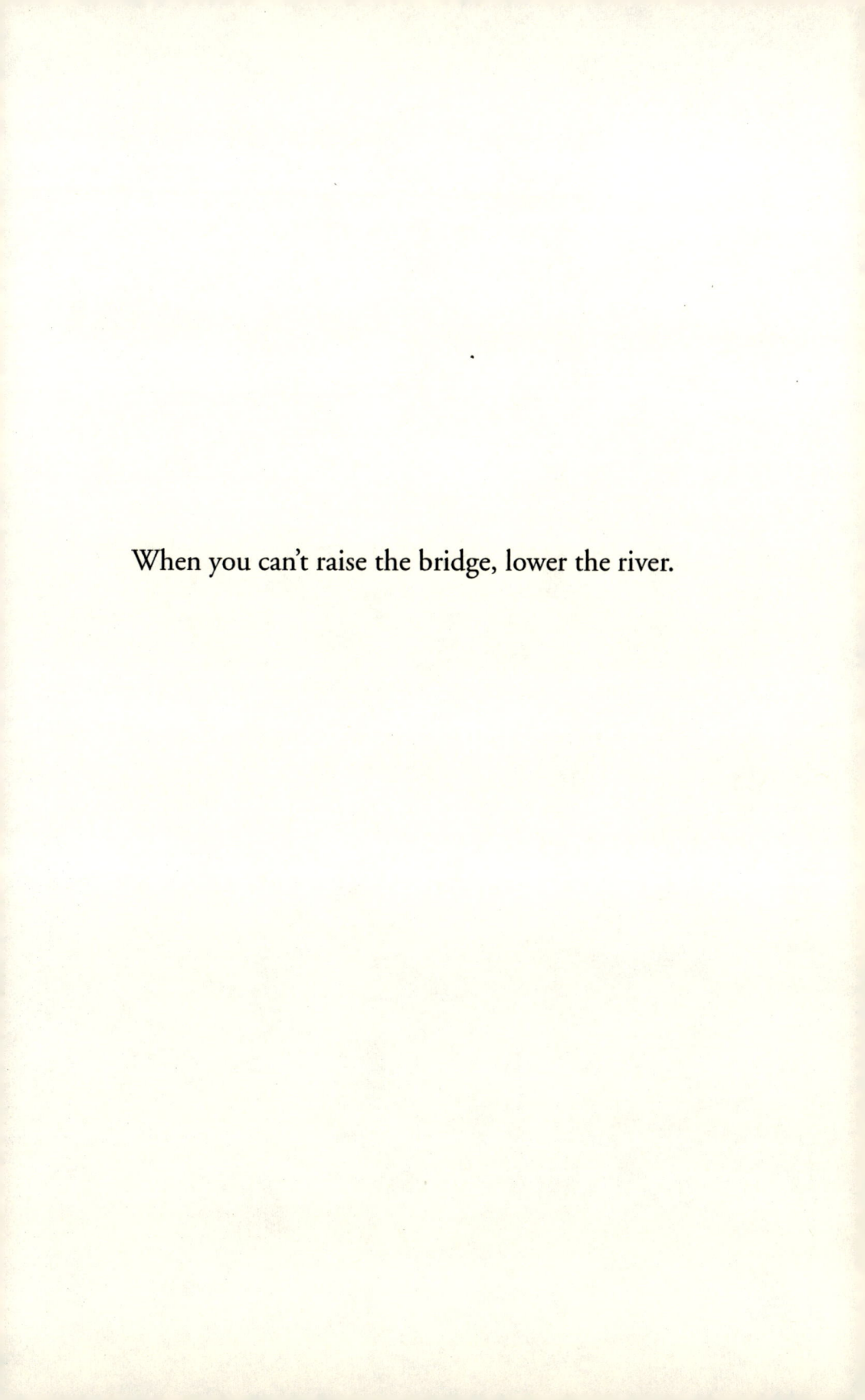

Contents

Foreword xi
Creatine Reduction Self-help Guide 1
    Creatine vs. Creatinine, or Bio-fuel vs. Bio-waste ..3
    Phosphorus, Potassium, and Sodium:
    What is meant by Low, Medium, and High? 10
    How to Use This Book 15
    Words to Know 18
    Handling and Storing Meat Safely 20
FRESH GROUND MEATS 25
    BEEF HAMBURGER (fresh) 27
    PORK (ground - fresh) 35
    TURKEY (ground - fresh) 39
FRESH ORGAN MEATS 45
    BEEF KIDNEY (fresh) 47
    BEEF LIVER (fresh) 52
FRESH CHICKEN 57
    CHICKEN STRIPS (fresh, skinned, chicken breast) 59

PROCESSED MEATS 65
    HAM (cured) 67
    WIENERS (pork) 70
CHEESE 73
    CHEESE (American Processed Cheese - slices) . . .75
MY PERSONAL DIETARY INSTRUCTIONS 79
MY DIETITIAN'S RECOMMENDATIONS 80
ADDITIONAL NOTES 81
Conclusions 83
About the Author 85
References 87

Foreword

Creatine, a component of meat, is one of the uremic toxins thought to contribute to the cycle of nausea, vomiting and anorexia in patients with kidney disease. This is a dilemma for these patients since their protein requirements are increased and meat intake is encouraged. Wendy Lou Jones, through exhaustive research, has created a unique and creative tool to help break this cycle while maintaining adequate protein intake to prevent malnutrition.

This text is beautifully written and very easy to understand. Ms. Jones has addressed many important issues including critical food safety tips and the background information needed to understand the concepts of creatine removal. The techniques are well detailed and simple to follow. The perfection of these techniques, with particular attention to taste and quality of the meat, is very impressive.

By applying the techniques outlined in this text, patients with kidney disease can achieve a bio-waste level comparable to a vegetarian diet while enjoying the meat taste. This could be a very important improvement in the diet for kidney disease and contribute to improving their symptoms. Working closely with members of the healthcare team, this important work offers patients with kidney disease more flexibility and potential for improved tolerance of the diet. Wendy Lou Jones' research in this, previously uncharted, area could prove to be essential in improving the outcomes of patients with kidney disease.

Cathi J. Martin, RD, CSR, LDN

This work was supported by a grant
from Royal Knight Research.

Creatine Reduction Self-help Guide

Dietary Creatine Reduction Self-help Guide for People with Kidney Impairment

CREATINE VS. CREATININE, OR BIO-FUEL VS. BIO-WASTE

Creatine – you may have seen it on the shelf, or read that some bodybuilders use it in the hopes of building bigger muscles. And while some athletes feel that maintaining a higher than normal physiological level of creatine gives their body that performance "edge", the only thing that a higher than normal physiological level of creati**nine** is associated with is renal (kidney) dysfunction, or failure.

If creatine and creatinine are so intricately related, why should a simple letter exchange—"e" to "**ine**"—make a physiological excess of this substance an indication of something so bad?

What is creatine? What is creatinine?
Simply put, creatine represents bio-fuel, a physiologically essential nitrogenous compound. When creatine combines with phosphorus, creatine-phosphate forms a metabolically essential high-energy phosphate. Creatinine, on the other hand, can be thought of as the "spent fuel" or bio-waste.

Creatine is an essential constituent of all muscle tissue (including the heart). Since its discovery in 1832, creatine has been shown to exist in high concentrations in all muscles involved in strenuous work (legs [calf, thigh, hip], arms, chest, back). More than 95% of the total creatine content is stored in the skeletal muscles, of this 1/3 is in its free form (Balsom, et al. 1994).

Between 10 - 30% of creatinine generated in the human body is derived from ingestion of creatine and creatinine found in various animal flesh (meats) (Levey, et al. 1988). While trace amounts of creatine has been found in milk (whole), cheese, and some plant matter, meat is the main source of exogenous (external) creatine(s) for most humans. In the absence of exogenous creatine (as exists in a totally vegetarian diet), creatine is created via endogenous (internal) synthesis (Delanghe, et al. 1989). The rate of turnover (creatine-creatinine) in the adult human body has been estimated to be around 1.6% per day (Hoogwerf, et al. 1986).

Endogenous creatine synthesis occurs outside of the muscle, primarily from the three precursor amino acids: arginine, glycine and methionine (Balsom, et al. 1994; Delanghe, et al. 1989). Enzymes involved in creatine synthesis are located in the liver, kidneys and pancreas. Synthesis begins with the transfer of amidine group from arginine to glycine (transamidination) to form guanidinoacetate and ornithine. The formation of creatine occurs via an irreversible addition of a methyl group from adenosylmethionine (Balsom, et al. 1994). Once synthesis is complete, creatine is transported back into the muscle via the bloodstream. While in the bloodstream, the creatine molecule is acted upon by enzymes that catalyze the transfer of phosphates, ultimately releasing its reactive phosphate moiety. This phosphate moiety goes on to interact with adenosine diphosphate, producing a very high-energy molecule called adenosine triphosphate or ATP.

Presently, more than a quarter of a million people in the United States are undergoing long-term dialysis because of end stage renal disease (ESRD) (Anonymous, 1998). The human kidney is responsible for influencing or acting upon a myriad of biological systems (red blood cell production, vitamin-D activation, parathyroid hormone, etc.). Two of the many life-sustaining functions kidneys perform are the regulation of physiological creatinine and mineral concentrations. As kidney failure escalates, the concentrations of many physiological minerals (phosphorus, potassium, and sodium), as well as nitrogenous waste, raise steadily until dialysis becomes necessary to curb symptomatic toxic uremia. While it has not definitively been established that creatinine, in and of itself, is cellularly toxic, it is a surrogate marker of small molecular weight nitrogenous uremic toxins, and in itself contributes to creatinine overload.

Certain dietary choices that a patient may make can add to the overall negative impact on their health. These choices include eating an excess amount of meat (outside of their consumption restrictions), eating the majority of their meat with a charred or blackened surface, as well as including a large amount of meat gravies in the diet. All of this can cause creatinine, and nitrogenous wastes (as well as excess minerals) to accumulate in higher concentrations, between dialysis sessions, than can be adequately removed during a single treatment period.

To date, only a few scientific authors have explored creatine removal from meat from a non-dialysis context. Jacobsen (et al. 1979) was able to demonstrate that the creatine concentration of minced chunks of goulash beef (approximately 1-inch cubes) declined to approximately half its original value after being subjected to a boiling water bath for as long as 180 minutes. Analysis of the water showed that its creatinine content had increased more than four-fold during the same period. No mention was made of the taste or texture of the goulash beef after subjecting it to such rigorous cooking.

Felton (et al. 1994) reported that the overall creatine content of ground beef hamburger could be reduced approximately 43% by subjecting it to microwave pre-cooking alone. Creatine losses were accounted for by analysis of the meat juice drippings.

Heat has been found to play a major role in the formation of creatinine from creatine. Meat, subjected to normal frying or broiling temperatures, produced gravy which contained as much as four times the amount of creatine, and more than 13 times the amount of creatinine, as found in raw beef (Jägerstad, et al. 1991).

The effects of dietary choices on serum creatinine levels in healthy individuals have been reported sporadically throughout literature. Ingesting cooked beef (but not raw beef) was found to causes a rapid, and substantial, postprandial (following a meal) rise in serum creatinine, peaking between 1.5 and 3 hours after ingestion (Jacobsen, et al. 1979). Consuming boiled beef, along with the water in which it was boiled, produced a much more dramatic, and pronounced, increase compared to frying alone. The same results were observed when equal gram quantities of pork were substituted for beef, or when beet and pork were mixed. In normal individuals, this temporary increase has not been associated with any negative health impact. Mayersohn (et al. 1983), using normal volunteers, reported a 52% increase in creatinine production within three hours after ingesting a single 225-gram meal of cooked meat. In addition, a postprandial elevation declines slowly, and can even remain elevated as long as 10 hours after ingestion in otherwise normal individuals (Jacobsen, et al. 1979).

When renal function is compromised, creatinine (as well as other minerals and nitrogenous waste) can not be eliminated fast enough to reduce the previous meal's load before the next is ingested. Consequently, each meal contributes to a preexisting elevated systemic load. This creates a precarious nutritional paradox. Meat provides essential protein – it is also the average renal patient's major source of dietary creatinine (and phosphorus). Excess phosphorus (in the presence of excess calcium) creates a negative impact, not only on the bones, but also on the entire circulatory system itself.

In an attempt to reduce creatinine (and phosphorus) build up, strict meat consumption restrictions are usually imposed – many times with mixed success. But, because meat is traditionally a very important part of the average American diet, any attempt to restrict its consumption tends to lead to significant dietary noncompliance problems with patients who are suddenly thrust into totally new eating habits. Further misinterpretation of dietary instructions inevitably leads to nutritional deficit, and ultimately malnutrition, as a cycle of toxemia related nausea ensues. This negative impact leads to an overall increase in the number of "sick days", both pre and post dialysis as well as a significant reduction in the patient's perception of wellbeing and quality of life. Prolonged poor nutrition ultimately contributes to increased patient morbidity and a rise in dialysis center mortality rates (Acchiardo, et al.1983; Maiorca, et al. 1995). It has been said that improving and managing personal nutrition is the most important "self help" area in which the patient can, individually, have the greatest influence.

The objective of this book is to provide the renal dietitian, renal patient and their renal health partners with a clear, easy to understand and follow, consumer friendly instructions on how to carry out the simplest, yet most efficacious, creatine and mineral reduction procedures. These procedures are applicable to several common dietary selections of meat as well as cheese. In addition to creatine reduction information, recipe tips for each item so treated, are provided at the ends of each food selection.

Consuming a total dietary selection of creatine reduced meats is expected to have a positive impact on the renal patients nutritional profile, as well as their problematic serum creatinine values. In an unpublished study conducted by this author, renal and control volunteer's creatinine levels were measured, both pre- and after a ten day period in which the volunteers consumed only creatine reduced (and demineralized) meats. Blood serum creatinine levels, from both control and renal volunteers, were positively impacted (to a greater extent in the renal impaired). Manipulating dietary creatine levels can positively influence blood serum creatinine levels (Jones, 2001).

phosphorus, potassium and sodium removal procedures for an entire dietary range of more than 50 foods selections are fully covered in the book: *"What you need to know about Healthy Living With Demineralization - Food demineralization instructions for people with kidney impairment"* (expected in spring of 2002) by Wendy Lou Jones, forward by Beth McQuiston, MS, RD, LD.

Phosphorus, Potassium, and Sodium: What is meant by Low, Medium, and High?

Regulation of serum creatinine concentration is just one of many important life-sustaining functions kidneys must perform. As kidney function declines, maintaining the correct internal balance of **phosphorus, potassium**, and **sodium** becomes more difficult to regulate as well. Unfortunately, meats and cheese contain an overabundance of at least one or more of these minerals. Unrestricted consumption of such mineral laden foods can cause physiological mineral imbalance (especially excess in potassium), that can lead to potentially dangerous, and even life threatening, health problems. It is, therefore, important that you know the amount of phosphorus, potassium, and sodium, per serving, of the foods you are about to prepare.

The following are definitions for low, medium and high mineral contents as they are used in this book.

phosphorus (P)
Neither the National Kidney Foundation, nor the American Dietetic Association have specified absolute low, medium, or high range guidelines for phosphorus per serving for kidney patients. With the exception of prepackaged foods, large concentrations of phosphorus are found primarily in meats, legumes/nuts, and dairy products. These foods supply essential protein and can not be eliminated from the diet. The National Kidney Foundation – Dialysis Outcomes Quality Initiative (NKF-DOQI) has made specific recommendations concerning protein – about1.2 grams per kilogram of body weight/day for hemodialysis patients (DOQI (a), 2000), and 1.2 – 1.3 grams per kilogram of body weight/day for chronic peritoneal dialysis (CPD).(DOQI (b), 2000) Based on an average concentration of 14 – 17 mg of phosphorus per gram of protein, a general rule of thumb for the amount of phosphorus found in a diet which contains about 1.2 grams of protein/kg body weight, would reasonably be:
For a 60kg person (132lb) = 1092—1326 mg of phosphorus/day;
For a 70kg person (154lb) = 1274—1547 mg phosphorus/day;
For an 80kg person (176lb) = 1456—1768 mg phosphorus/day.

Unfortunately, when little or no kidney function remains, many patients find it virtually impossible to maintain a normal, or even near normal, blood phosphorus level, consuming this amount of dietary phosphorus, without substantial use of phosphate binders. The need for proper nutrition usually makes a low physiological phosphorus goal unattainable.

One of the many benefits to demineralizing food is that much lower nutritional phosphorus levels can be achieved without sacrificing needed protein.

Based on the nutritional phosphorus reduction potential achievable by using the creatine reduction procedures listed in this book, this author has calculated *prospective* low, medium, and high ranges for the food selections tested. It is understood that these ranges are **only** intended for use within the context of this book.

(a) *Low*: 0 - 110 mg or less per serving
(b) *Medium*: 111 - 200 mg per serving
   High: 201 mg per serving and up.

The above calculations were based on a daily phosphorus limit of 1000 mg, distributed across 3 meals per day (with 2 or 3 phosphorus items per meal) in the following calculation:

(a) 110 mg of P per each 100 gram item x 3 items per meal x 3 meals/day
   = less than 1000 mg of phosphorus/day (about 990 mg of P)

(b) 200 mg of P per each 100 gram item x 2 items per meal x 3 meals/day
   = more than 1000 mg of phosphorus (about 1200 mg of P)

(To illustrate a point—performing a 30-minute creatine reduction procedure on beef hamburger will reduce the phosphorus content an average of more than 40%, placing it in the *low* phosphorus category, *according to this book*. An individual would theoretically have to consume more than 1400 grams [about 50 ounces, or more then 3 lb.] of demineralized hamburger [containing roughly 325 - 350 grams of protein], in order to have consumed 1000 mg of phosphorus.)

Potassium (K)
Existing guidelines for hemodialysis patients generally recommend limiting potassium ingestion (approximately 60 - 70 milliequivalents (mEq) or about 2,300 to 2,700 mg per day) (Ahmed, et al., 1997), depending upon individualized medical restrictions. The following defined low, medium, and high values for potassium per serving are currently in use for **hemodialysis** patients:

Low: 0 – 100 mg per serving
Medium: 101 – 200 mg per serving
High: 201 – 350 mg per serving

Sodium (Na)
Currently, hemodialysis patients are usually told to limit sodium intake to between 2 – 3 grams or 2000 – 3000 mg per day, depending upon individualized medical restrictions. The govern-

ment nutrition labeling guidelines (Anonymous, 1998) specify that food with less than:
5mg of sodium per serving can be labeled "**sodium-free**",
35 mg or less per serving - "**very-low-sodium**",
less than 140 mg of sodium per serving - "**low-sodium**".

The National Renal Diet patient education and meal planning booklets have labeled any foods, with more than 250 mg of sodium, with a saltshaker symbol *suggesting* "high sodium". While professional renal nutrition guidelines for sodium, in use today, do not state defined low, or medium classifications for this mineral, using the government nutrition labeling guidelines and the National Renal Diet patient education information, this author has ascribed *prospective* low, medium, and high *ranges*. It is understood that these ranges are intended for use **only** within the context of this book

Low: 0 – 140 mg per serving
Medium: 141 – 249 mg per serving
High: 250 mg or more per serving

Remember that the minerals phosphorus, potassium, and sodium, found in everyday foods aren't bad – indeed, the body could not survive, or continue to function, in their complete absence. But, there is a reasonably narrow metabolic mineral range, which is considered to be normal. Just as the absence of one or more of these minerals would prove highly detrimental, an imbalance, and/or an excess of one or more of these minerals can also lead to a potentially life-threatening situation.

How to Use This Book

The information presented in this work is based on meat creatine and mineral reduction data from several studies conducted by the author. Each food item is treated as follows:

1. The foods selection is listed at the top of each page:
BEEF HAMBURGER (fresh)

2. The approximate original creatine content
    per 100 grams (about 3 1/2 ounce) serving,
   without special preprocessing and after frying is listed below:
    440 mg of Creatine

3. The original mineral content per serving for
    one or more of the target minerals, before processing,
    (sodium [Na], potassium [K], phosphorus [P]),
    is displayed in milligrams:

K	P	Na
216 mg	123 mg	44 mg

4. The approximate creatine concentration remaining and creatine reduction potential of a specific procedure, as well as the remaining target mineral concentration and mineral reduction potential:

Procedure A   **Reduction Potential**
14 mg of Creatine   96%
Minerals Remaining and Reduction Potential

K	P	Na	K	P	Na
36 mg	70 mg	9 mg	83%	43%	80%

5. Processing instructions including any specific special notation.
6. Post processing recipe suggestions.

The creatine content data, cited in this book, was obtained from several creatine reduction studies in which food samples, thus processed, were analyzed at Eurofins Scientific Inc., a US analytical testing facility. Demineralization data, cited in this book, was obtained from food samples tested at Midwest Laboratories, Inc., an USDA food testing laboratory in Omaha, NE.

It should be noted that there is no single 'standard' creatine or mineral concentration for any meat. While literature provides a generalized species value, the original creatine (and mineral) content of a selection of meat depends largely upon a number of factors, including whether the selection came from muscle or non-muscle (organ) meat, and the type of animal being utilized.

Creatine content has been shown to vary significantly between animal species and flesh type (Vikse and Joner, 1993).

Vikse was able to demonstrate that 50 gram portions of muscle meat, sampled from 16 different meat animals, each produced different concentrations of creatine(s). Of the 16 different species tested, domestic rabbit, followed by seal, deer, beef, pork, sheep, horse, and reindeer consistently gave the highest level of creatine(s) .

The creatine content for several traditional American selections of fish and meat are: cod (3 g/kg), herring (6.5-10 g/kg), salmon (4.5g/kg), tuna (4g/kg), beef hamburger (4.5g/kg), and pork (5g/kg). Over all, irrespective of the species sampled (domestic or wild), researchers have confirmed, muscle meats contain the highest amounts of creatine and creatinine while organ meats (liver and kidney) contain the lowest.

Because of this wide variation, all creatine and mineral values, cited in this book, should be viewed as the contents **only** for the food sample that was tested. The 100-gram beef hamburger flesh that you process for creatine/ mineral removal may have slightly more or less creatine/mineral load than is listed in this book. However, regardless of your meat selections initial creatine/mineral concentration, if you are carrying out the processing procedure, exactly as described for that selection, you can reasonably expect the percent of creatine/mineral lost to closely approximate that shown in this book

Words to Know

The following words will be used in relation to creatine and mineral content as well as the reduction processes described in this book.

Creatine:
A physiologically essential, high-energy phosphate, nitrogenous compound.

Creatinine:
A waste product formed from the metabolism of creatine.

Creation Reduction:
The removal of creatine (and minerals) from a substance. In this book, creatine reduction is accomplished by exposing a food selection to water at various temperatures for various time periods.

Gram (g):
A unit of weight. A 100-gram sample is approximately equal to 3.5 ounces, or a standard serving size for most foods.

K: A shorthand chemical symbol for potassium.

Milligram (mg):
A unit of weight equaling 1/1000 of a gram. 1000 milligrams is equal to 1 gram. A serving size, as listed in this book, is 100 grams.

Na: A shorthand chemical symbol for sodium.

P: A shorthand chemical symbol for phosphorus.

Arginine, Glycine and Methionine:
Creatine synthesis occurs primarily from these three precursor amino acids.

Endogenous Creatine Synthesis:
The internal synthesis of creatine from amino acids.

Postprandial Creatinine Elevation:
Creatinine elevation which occurs after a meat meal.

HANDLING AND STORING MEAT SAFELY

Improper food handling and storage can lead to food poisoning! It is absolutely essential that all food handling, processing, and storage procedures be carried out with clean hands, on a clean surface, using clean food preparation utensils. Do not reuse utensils later on in the process without washing them first. To do so can lead to cross contamination.

If you are beginning with frozen meats, be sure to defrost it in the refrigerator overnight, not on the counter at room temperature! Improperly defrosted meat can lead to food poisoning. For faster thawing, you can place a package of frozen food in a watertight plastic bag submerged under cold water. Note – cheese is the only exception to the "no-countertop thawing" rule. Frozen cheese can be thawed on the counter top until it is soft enough to slice.

Upon opening any package, check all food for any 'off' smell, color, or abnormal appearance. Do not rely on your sense of smell alone. **Tasting spoiled, raw meat can prove hazardous to**

your health! Discard any outdated foods without tasting because they can harbor deadly bacteria.

Keeping foods clean is as easy as frequent hand washing. Always soap up and scrub before touching raw meat. And, don't "carry" hidden contamination – always remember to use a clean cloth to dry your hands. Don't use that same cloth to periodically wipe your meat soiled hands then touch the meat again and again. This will only carry potential bacterial contamination from your initial foodstuff to your working area.

When working with raw meat and poultry, DO wash hands often, as well as counters, and utensils, in HOT soapy water, between each recipe step. Even a small amount of bacteria can prove dangerous. NEVER put cooked meat or poultry on the same plate that held the raw food.

Be sure to finish cooking all foods before consuming them. Check for "pinkness" before you finish cooking. If the meat is still pink, it is underdone and could harbor bacteria. Also, do not partially cook food, stop, then at a later period (i.e. hours or days later) "finish" the cooking process. If left long enough, bacteria will grow before the second cooking. Discard any cooked or chilled food that has been left out on the counter for more than two hours.

Once foods are cooked, be sure to keep hot foods hot. Eat all food during a single meal or refrigerate at once. Store leftovers in the refrigerator as soon as possible after eating. Do not allow food to cool on the counter. In order to safely inhibit bacterial growth, keep your refrigerator at 40ºF, and your freezer at 0ºF or less. This will insure food safety.

When preparing food for storage, use strong moisture proof materials such as heavy plastic (i.e. freezer grade) aluminum foil, freezer paper, intact freezer bags, freezer wrap, or freezer containers. Keep cooked meat or poultry away from any equipment or utensils that have been in contact with raw meat or poultry until they have been properly washed. If you have purchased additional meat and poultry, freeze or chill meat and poultry in the store's original package. If you are planning to store your meat for a longer period of time (i.e. several months), place the wrapped meat in a freezer bag before freezing.

You can store processed meat and cheese approximately 3 to 4 months in the freezer.

Using the procedures listed in the following pages of this text, this author has safely reduced the creatine and mineral content from meat, poultry, and cheese.

Note, ground meat, or pre-processed meat (i.e. lunched meats, hot dogs, etc.) may contain more bacteria than a solid chunk of meat, depending upon how it was handled during processing at the plant. Some of the meats, listed in this guide, are subjected to a 30-minute warm-water (approximately 100ºF) creatine reduction procedure. Exposing meat to warm water will cause bacteria to multiply. So, before beginning any creatine reduction procedure, check the meat you are intending to use and be absolutely certain that it is not already spoiled (**when in doubt – throw it out!**). Be sure to discard any meat that has reached the expiration date, regardless of what you do (or don't) smell.

Store all creatine-reduced processed foods, not immediately eaten, in the refrigerator. Foods thus processed spoil very quickly – including cheese. Be sure to thoroughly cook and eat, or with in 24 hours, freeze all creatine-reduced foods (cheese is the only exception to the freezing rule). Freezing will prevent spoilage, allowing you to process large batches of food and keep it for later use

FRESH GROUND MEATS

After processing, it is normal for all meats to appear substantially lighter in color. This color change happens because most of the meat blood is removed during processing. The loss of meat tissue blood does not in any way mean that the meat is "bad". It is perfectly **OK** to eat meat that has little or no blood associated with it.

BEEF HAMBURGER (FRESH)

Approximate creatine and mineral concentration per 100 grams (about 3 1/2 ounces) of beef hamburger meat, without special processing, and after frying:
    440 mg of Creatine
K – 216 mg P – 123 mg Na – 44 mg

Approximate creatine and mineral content remaining in 100 grams of beef hamburger meat, after meat has been prepared according to **Procedure A or B:**

Procedure A	**Reduction Potential**
14 mg of Creatine	96%

Minerals Remaining and Reduction Potential

K	P	Na	K	P	Na
36 mg	70 mg	9 mg	83%	43%	80%

Procedure B   **Reduction Potential**
3 mg of Creatine   >99%

Processing Instructions:
(Be sure to follow safe meat handling and storage procedures at all times!)

Procedure A—

1. Remove fresh ground beef hamburger from its package and discard the package. Crumble meat into a kitchen strainer. Rinse under cold running water for 15 – 20 seconds.
2. Place up to 1 pound of rinsed hamburger in a minimum of 1 liter of warm tap water (approximately 100°F), disperse meat by briefly stirring vigorously.
3. Allow meat to stand for a one half hour on the counter.
4. Drain meat in a clean kitchen colander or sieve*—**do not keep or use the water, it contains creatine/creatinine and excess minerals!**

This ends processing **Procedure A.** You may stop here and cook your meat.

If you plan to fry your meat, be sure to place the drained meat on a small stack of paper towels, and blot off excess moisture before frying, to avoid spattering.

    Add spices and other ingredients as desired, mix thoroughly before forming patties. This author recommends using low heat for frying in order to avoid charring or toughening your meat.

*NOTE - If you wish to lower the creatine content of the meat further, before it is eaten, do not add spices or cook, but proceed directly from **step 4** to **Procedure B.**

Procedure B—
1. Placed the meat from **Step 4 (Procedure A)** into a minimum of 1 liter of water heated to between 170 - 180°F (light simmer - not boiling!).
2. Stir for approximately three minutes.
3. Drain into a clean colander or sieve which has not come in contact with raw meat—**do not keep or use this water, it contains creatine/creatinine and excess minerals!**
4. Blot dry on a small stack of paper towels and serve.

Meat processed through **Procedure B** is cooked and will require the use of a binding material (i.e., addition of egg or gluten) in order to form it into patties or hold a specific shape, such as for a meat loaf. Alternately, hamburger processed through **Procedure B** can be used as crumbles in a salad, on a sandwich, or it can be seasoned and briefly fried (low heat) to give it that special 'fry' taste.

Be sure to refrigerate any unused processed meat (from **Procedure A** or **B**) immediately. Use within 24 hours. Alternately, meat may be frozen for later use.

Recipe Tips for After Processing
1) After processing (**Procedure A**) is complete, hamburger can be formed into patties to fry on low to medium heat. This author recommends using no trans fatty acids (and low sodium) margarine. Served with your favorite condiments.

2) Hamburger crumbles (from **Procedure A or B**) can be heated in no trans-fatty acid (and low sodium) margarine and made into barbecues.

Best Burger B.B.Q. Sauce
Ingredients:
1 small bottle of ketchup
2 packed tbls brown sugar
¼ cup of white corn syrup
1 tsp prepared mustard
3 drops of hickory smoke (or to taste)
1 tbls molasses (any kind)

In order to dissolve the brown sugar and meld the flavors, simmered (on low heat) for several minutes while stirring. Pour the mixture into a bottle and store any excess in the refrigerator for later use.

Home Made Meat Loaf (meat from Procedure A)
Ingredients:
1 lb hamburger
1 cup of bread crumbles (fine)
1 medium onion minced (fine)

3 egg whites
¼ cup of B.B.Q. sauce
1/8 tsp Mrs. Dash
Cook, as per your recipe, in a microwave or conventional oven.

Beef and No-Yoke Noodle Dish
Ingredients:
1-lb of processed beef (**Procedure A**)
1–1/2 cups of no yolk noodles
water
1 (15-oz) can of onion soup
Worcestershire sauce (a dash)

Form meatballs. Place meat in a 2-quart microwave dish. Add onion soup, sufficient water to cook the noodles, and Worcestershire sauce. Mix well and microwave on high, stirring occasionally. Check during cooking to see if extra water is needed. When noodles are hydrated and soft, cover and let stand for 10 minutes. Be sure to refrigerate any unused portion.

To reheat: Use a vented microwave cover or microwave plastic wrap. Stir intermittently during microwaving. Microwave until sufficiently hot. Let beef casserole stand, covered, 1 minute before serving.

Timely Tacos
Ingredients:
Tacos shells
1-lb of processed (**Procedure B**) beef hamburger
tomatoes
onions
lettuce
(processed) cheese
olives

Assemble the ingredients. Layer ingredients in the shell, add mayonnaise or Ketchup, or B.B.Q. sauce to taste. Serve hot or cold. Alternately, ingredient may be layered on a burrito and placed into the microwave. Microwave on high until hot.

Be sure to refrigerate any unused portion as soon as the meal is finished. Extra Tacos (or burrito) may be frozen and reheated for a later meal.

Stuffed "Peppy" Peppers
Ingredients:
1-lb of processed (**Procedure B**) beef
6-large hollowed out peppers (any color)
2 tbs of no trans fatty acids margarine
Tomato juice
A dash of B.B.Q. sauce or Tabasco sauce (if desired)

Mix ingredients and place in hollowed out peppers. Microwave on high until peppers are soft. Allow microwaved food to stand 1 minute before serving. Author's Hint – a small dash of Tabasco sauce goes along way!

Home-Made Party Pizza
Ingredients:
1-lb of processed (**Procedure B**) beef hamburger or pork burger
2 Tortilla shells per pizza (8" size)
diced tomatoes
diced onions
diced peppers (green or red)
(processed) cheese
minced olives
anchovies (optional)
tomato sauce or pizza sauce
artichoke hearts
baby corn cobs

Assemble ingredients. Place processed cheese between the two shells. Add pizza sauce, cheese, and other ingredients on top. Top mix with more (processed) cheese, and microwave on several thickness of paper toweling. Pizza is done when cheese begins to melt. Be sure to refrigerate any unused portion. Consume within 24 hours if not frozen.

Spiffy Spaghetti—Beef Dish
Ingredients:
1-lb of beef hamburger, formed into meatballs (**Procedure A**), or as crumbles (**Procedure B**)
½ cup of finely chopped onions,
½ cup finely chopped peppers
1 can of 4 cheese spaghetti sauce
1 to 2 bay leaves
cooked spaghetti
Processed cheese

Cook the spaghetti according to the direction on the package. In a separate pan, place the other ingredients and cook slowly until the beef and vegetables are tender. Serve separately or mixture and spaghetti can be combined prior to serving. Chunk additional (processed) cheese on top of the spaghetti if desired. For a dash of color, try sprinkling diced red and yellow peppers on top of the spaghetti, or garnishing with a little parley.

PORK (GROUND - FRESH)

Approximate creatine and mineral concentration per 100 grams (about 3 1/2 ounces) of ground pork meat, without special processing, and after frying:

490 mg of Creatine
K – 172 mg P – 196 mg

Approximate creatine and mineral content remaining in 100 grams of ground pork meat, after meat has been prepared according to **Procedure A or B**:

Procedure A   Reduction Potential
74 mg of Creatine   85%
Minerals Remaining and Reduction Potential
K	P	K	P
57 mg	80 mg	67%	59%

Procedure B   Reduction Potential
10 mg of Creatine   98%

Processing Instructions:
(Be sure to follow safe meat handling and storage procedures at all times!)

Procedure A—
1. Remove fresh ground (unseasoned) pork from its package and discard the package. Crumble pork into a clean kitchen strainer. Rinse under cold running water for 15 – 20 seconds.
2. Place up to 1 pound of rinsed ground pork in a minimum of 1 liter of warm tap water (approximately 100°F), disperse meat by briefly stirring vigorously.
3. Allowed meat to stand for a one half hour on the counter.
4. Drain meat in a clean kitchen colander or sieve*—**do not keep or use the water, it contains creatine/creatinine and excess minerals!**

This ends processing **Procedure A.** You may stop here and cook your meat.

If you plan to fry your meat, be sure to place the drained meat on a small stack of paper towels, and blot off excess moisture before frying to avoid spattering.

Add spices and other ingredients as desired, mix thoroughly before forming patties. This author recommends using low heat for frying in order to avoid charring or toughening your meat.

*NOTE - If you wish to lower the creatine content of the meat further, before it is eaten, do not add spices or cook, but proceed directly from **step 4** to **Procedure B.**

Procedure B—
1. Placed the meat from **Step 4 (Procedure A)** into a minimum of 1 liter of water heated to between 170 - 180°F (light simmer - not boiling!).
2. Stir for approximately three minutes.
3. Drain into a clean colander or sieve—**do not keep or use the water, it contains creatine/creatinine and excess minerals!**
4. Blot dry on a small stack of paper towels and serve.

Meat processed through **Procedure B** is cooked and will require the use of a binding material (i.e., addition of egg or gluten) in order to form it into patties or hold a specific shape, such as for a meat loaf. Alternately, ground pork processed through **Procedure B** can be used as crumbles in a salad, on a sandwich, or it can be seasoned and briefly fried (low heat) to give it that special 'fry' taste.

Be sure to refrigerate any unused processed meat (from **Procedure A or B**) immediately. Use within 24 hours or meat may also be frozen for later use.

Recipe Tips for After Processing
1) To make pork breakfast sausage (pork after **Procedure A**), season with your favorite spices, add 2 egg whites, form into

patties, fry on low heat. This author recommends using no trans fatty acids (and low sodium) margarine. Serve with fried or scrambled egg whites and toast. One pound of pork sausage mix serves four.

2) Pork (**Procedure A** or **B**) can be used for flavoring for soups and vegetables. Be sure to thoroughly cook any pork/vegetable dish when using meat from Procedure A.

3) Press pork (after **Procedure A**), into meatballs, add spices to cook with sauerkraut, or in any noodle dishes.

TURKEY (GROUND - FRESH)

Approximate creatine and mineral concentration per 100 grams (about 3 1/2 ounces) of ground turkey meat, without special processing, and after frying:
    410 mg of Creatine
K – 245 mg   P – 208 mg

Approximate creatine and mineral content remaining in 100 grams of ground turkey meat, after meat has been prepared according to **Procedure A** or **B**:

Procedure A   Reduction Potential
92 mg of Creatine   78%
Minerals Remaining and Reduction Potential
K	P	K	P
45 mg	75 mg	82%	64%

Procedure B   Reduction Potential
11 mg of Creatine   97%

Processing Instructions:
(Be sure to follow safe meat handling and storage procedures at all times!)

Procedure A—

Note – If you grind your own turkey meat, be sure to skin it first. Creatine and minerals are not effectively removed from fat-laden meat.

1. Remove fresh ground turkey meat from its package and discard the package. Crumble poultry into a kitchen strainer. Rinse under **warm** (approximately 100°F) running water for 3 minutes.
2. Place up to 1 pound of rinsed ground turkey meat in a minimum of 1 liter of **cold** tap water, disperse meat by briefly stirring vigorously.
3. Allowed meat to stand for a one hour in the refrigerator – do not allow this meat to sit on the counter or remain at room temperature.
4. Drain meat in a clean kitchen colander or sieve*—**do not keep or use the water, it contains creatine/creatinine and excess minerals!**

This ends processing **Procedure A.** You may stop here and cook your meat.

If you plan to fry your meat, be sure to place the drained meat on a small stack of paper towels, and blot off excess moisture before frying, to avoid spattering.

Add spices and other ingredients as desired, mix thoroughly before forming patties. This author recommends using low heat for frying in order to avoid charring or toughening your meat.

*NOTE - If you wish to lower the creatine content of the meat further, before it is eaten, do not add spices or cook, but proceed directly from **step** 4 to **Procedure B.**

Procedure B—
1. Placed the meat from **Step 4 (Procedure A)** into a minimum of 1 liter of water heated to between 170 - 180°F (light simmer - not boiling!).
2. Stir for approximately three minutes.
3. Drain into a clean colander or sieve—**do not keep or use the water, it contains creatine/creatinine and excess minerals!**
4. Blot dry on a small stack of paper towels and serve.

Meat processed through **Procedure B** is cooked and will require the use of a binding material (i.e., addition of egg or gluten) in order to form it into patties or hold a specific shape, such as for a meat loaf. Turkey burger processed through **Procedure B** can be used as crumbles in a salad, on a sandwich, or it can be seasoned and briefly fried (low heat) to give it that special 'fry' taste.

Be sure to refrigerate any unused processed meat (from **Procedure A or B**) immediately. Use within 24 hours, or meat may be frozen for later use.

Recipe Tips for After Processing

Ground turkey (after **Procedure A** or **B**) is very good seasoned with sage, poultry seasoning, or thyme to suit your taste. Add 2 egg whites and a little Mrs. Dash, form into patties and fry on low to medium heat. This author recommends using a small amount of no trans fatty acids (and low sodium) margarine.

Quick Turkey Rice
Ingredients:
Turkey (Procedure A) spiced as follows:
>Poultry seasoning
>Sage
>Mrs. Dash (if desired)
>Black pepper (if desired)

Form into balls – approximately 1 inch in diameter.

Cook instant rice (according to instructions) until almost done. Then place in an oven/microwave safe dish and add one small can of mushroom soupe and meatballs. Cook in the oven (at 325°F or 350°F) or in the microwave until meat is done.

Tom-Turkey Spaghetti Dish
Ingredients:
1-lb of turkey, formed into meatballs (**Procedure A**), or as crumbles (**Procedure B**)
½ cup of finely chopped onions,
½ cup finely chopped peppers
1 can of 4 cheese spaghetti sauce

1 to 2 bay leaves
cooked spaghetti
Processed cheese

Cook the spaghetti according to the direction on the package. In a separate pan, place the other ingredients and cook slowly until the turkey and vegetables are done. Serve separately or combine the sauce and spaghetti prior to serving. Chunk additional (processed) cheese on top of the spaghetti if desired. For a dash of color, try sprinkling diced red and yellow peppers on top of the spaghetti, or garnishing with a little parley.

Gobbling-Good Stuffed Peppers
Ingredients:
1-lb of processed (**Procedure B**) Turkey
6-large hollowed out peppers (any color)
2 tbs of no trans fatty acids margarine
Tomato juice
A dash of B.B.Q. sauce or Tabasco sauce (if desired)

Mix ingredient and place in hollowed out peppers. Microwave on high until the peppers are soft. Allow microwaved food to stand 1 minute before serving. Authors Hint – a small dash of Tabasco sauce goes a long way! For a touch of holiday color, try serving this mix with cranberry sauce or a small amount of orange marmalade.

FRESH ORGAN MEATS

After processing, it is normal for all meats to appear light in color. This color change happens because most of the meat blood is removed during processing. The loss of meat tissue blood does not, in any way, mean that the meat is "bad". It is perfectly **OK** to eat meat that has little or no blood associated with it.

BEEF KIDNEY (FRESH)

Approximate creatine and mineral concentration per 100 grams (about 3 1/2 ounces) of beef kidney, without special processing, and after frying:

36 mg of Creatine
K – 227   P – 233

Approximate creatine and mineral content remaining in 100 grams of sliced beef kidney after meat has been prepared according to **Procedure A or B**:

Procedure A   Reduction Potential
13 mg of Creatine   64%
Minerals Remaining and Reduction Potential
K	P	K	P
148 mg	213 mg	35%	9%

Procedure B   Reduction Potential
10 mg of Creatine   72%

Processing Instructions:
(Be sure to follow safe meat handling procedures at all times!)
Procedure A—
1. Remove fresh beef kidney from its package and discard the package. Slice kidney into strips approximately 1/4" to 1/8" inch in thickness.

NOTE - Whole meats must be sliced before creatine can be removed effectively.

2. Place sliced beef kidney in a kitchen strainer and rinse under cold running water for 15 – 20 seconds.
3. Place up to 1 pound of rinsed beef kidney slices in a minimum of 1 liter of warm tap water (approximately 100°F), disperse meat by briefly stirring vigorously;
4. Allowed meat to stand for a one half hour on the counter.
5. Drain meat in a clean kitchen colander or sieve*—**do not keep or use the water, it contains creatine/creatinine and excess minerals!**

This ends processing **Procedure A**. You may stop here and cook your meat.

If you plan to fry your meat, be sure to place the drained meat on a small stack of paper towels, and blot off excess moisture before frying, to avoid spattering.

Season as desired. If you intend to fry your meat, this author recommends using low heat for frying in order to avoid charring or toughening your meat.

*NOTE - If you wish to lower the creatine content of the kidney further, before it is eaten, proceed directly from **step** 4 to **Procedure B**. However, in the case of beef kidney, only a small reduction in total creatine content will result from this step.

Procedure B—
1. Placed the meat from **Step 4 (Procedure A)** into a minimum of 1 liter of water heated to between 170 - 180°F (light simmer - not boiling!).
2. Stir for approximately three to four minutes.
3. Drain into a clean colander or sieve—**do not keep or use the water, it contains creatine/creatinine and excess minerals!**
4. Blot dry on a small stack of paper towels and serve.

Meat processed through **Procedure B** is cooked (if the meat was sliced into 1/8" thickness). If the slice thickness was 1/4" thick or greater, check the doneness of the meat by slicing several of the thicker pieced in half and observe the center for 'pinkness'. Be sure to cook any underdone meat before eating.

Refrigerate any unused processed meat (from **Procedure A or B**) immediately. Use within 24 hours, or meat may be frozen for later use.

Recipe Tips for After Processing

1) Beef kidney is very good when cooked, or fried, slowly with onions. Treat beef kidney and onions as you would liver and onions. This author suggests that you use no trans fatty acids margarine for frying on low heat.

2) Simmer kidney in a medium amount of water until tender then drain. Using a hand grinder or a good food processor, and process until smooth. Add a small amount of Lite Miracle Whip salad dressing – just enough to make a pate or spread. Add ½ tsp of dry, or regular mustard, and ¼ cup of finely minced onion, and mix. If more moisture is needed use water or a few drops of lemon juice. This mix is great on bread or cracker, served as a lunch or as a snack.

3) Kidney and Rice Dish. This is a flavorful dish that can be made during any season.

Ingredients:
Beef Kidney from (Procedure A) spiced as follows:
>Poultry seasoning
>Sage
>Mrs. Dash (if desired)
>Black pepper (if desired)

Use approximately 1 lb of sliced kidney (Procedure A or B) for this dish.

Cook instant rice (according to instructions) until almost done. Then place in an oven/microwave safe dish and add one small can of mushroom soupe and kidney.

Cook in the oven (at 325°F or 350°F) or in the microwave until meat is done.

BEEF LIVER (FRESH)

Approximate creatine and mineral concentration per 100 grams (about 3 1/2 ounces) of beef liver, without special processing, and after frying:

    36 mg of Creatine
    K – 249   P - 284

Approximate creatine concentration remaining in 100 grams of sliced beef liver, after meat has been prepared according to **Procedure A or B**:

Procedure A   Reduction Potential
23 mg of Creatine   36%
Minerals Remaining and Reduction Potential

K	P	K	P
179 mg	240 mg	28%	>15%

Procedure B   Reduction Potential
10 mg of Creatine   72%

Processing Instructions:
(Be sure to follow safe meat handling procedures at all times!)

Procedure A—
1. Remove fresh beef liver from its package, discard the package and slice into strips approximately 1/4" to 1/8" inch in thickness.

NOTE - Whole meats must be sliced before creatine can be removed effectively.

2. Place sliced beef liver in a kitchen strainer and rinse under cold running water for 1- 3 minutes to remove excess blood.
3. Place up to 1 pound of rinsed beef liver slices in a minimum of 1 liter of warm tap water (approximately 100°F), disperse meat by briefly stirring vigorously.
4. Allowed meat to stand for a one half hour on the counter.
5. Drain meat in a clean kitchen colander or sieve*—**do not keep or use the water, it contains creatine/creatinine and excess minerals!**

This ends processing **Procedure A.** You may stop here and cook your meat.

If you plan to fry your meat, be sure to place the drained meat on a small stack of paper towels, and blot off excess moisture before frying, to avoid spattering. Season as desired. Liver fries fast, and this author recommends using low heat for frying in order to avoid over cooking and toughening your liver.

*NOTE - If you wish to lower the creatine content of the liver further, before it is eaten, proceed directly from **step** 4 to **Procedure B**.

Procedure B—
1. Placed the meat from **Step 4 (Procedure A)** into a minimum of 1 liter of water heated to between 170 - 180°F (light simmer - not boiling!).
2. Stir for approximately three to four minutes.
3. Drain into a clean colander or sieve—**do not keep or use the water, it contains creatine/creatinine and excess minerals!**
4. Blot dry on a small stack of paper towels and serve.

Meat processed through **Procedure B** is cooked (if the meat was sliced into 1/8" thickness). If the slice thickness was 1/4" thick or greater, check the doneness of the meat by slicing several of the thicker pieced in half and observe the center for 'pinkness'. Be sure to cook any underdone meat before eating.

Refrigerate any unused processed meat (from **Procedure A or B**) immediately. Use within 24 hours, or meat may be frozen for later use.

Recipe Tips for After Processing

After either processing procedure (**A** or **B**), liver is delicious cooked or fried with no trans fatty acids margarine and onions.

Lively Liver Pate: Use 1 lb of liver (**Procedure A or B**)

Simmer liver in a medium amount of water until done (if meat is being used from Procedure A), then drain. Using a hand grinder, or a good food processor, process until smooth. Add a small amount of Lite Miracle Whip salad dressing – just enough to make a pate or spread. Add ½ tsp of dry, or regular mustard, and ¼ cup of finely minced onion, and mix. If more moisture is needed use water or a few drops of lemon juice. This mix is great on bread or cracker (optional), served as a lunch or as a snack.

FRESH CHICKEN

Chicken will appear slightly lighter in color after processing, this is normal because tissue blood is lost during processing.

CHICKEN STRIPS
(FRESH, SKINNED, CHICKEN BREAST)

Approximate creatine and mineral concentration per 100 grams (about 3 1/2 ounces) of skinned chicken breast, without special processing, and after frying:

530 mg of Creatine
K – 190 mg   P – 184 mg

Approximate creatine and mineral content remaining in 100 grams of thinly sliced (1/8" to 1/4" inch thickness) and skinned chicken breast strips, after meat has been prepared according to **Procedure A** or **B**:

Procedure A   Reduction Potential
100 mg of Creatine   >80%

Minerals Remaning and Reduction Potential
  K   P   K   P
86 mg   96 mg   64%   48%

Procedure B   Reduction Potential
44 mg of Creatine   >90%

Processing Instructions:
(Be sure to follow safe meat handling procedures at all times!)
Procedure A—
NOTE - For easier slicing, this author recommends that the chicken be skinned, then lightly frozen before slicing.

1. Remove fresh **skinned** chicken breast from the freezer and slice into strips approximately 1/4" to 1/8" inch in thickness.
NOTE – Chicken must be skinned and the meat must be sliced before creatine and minerals can be effectively removed.
2. Place sliced chicken breast in a kitchen strainer and rinse under warm tap water (approximately 100°F) for 3 minutes.
3. Place up to 1 pound of rinsed chicken breast strips in a minimum of 1 liter of cold tap water, disperse meat by briefly stirring vigorously.
4. Allowed meat to stand for a one hour in the refrigerator.
5. Drain meat in a clean kitchen colander or sieve*—**do not keep or use the water, it contains creatine/creatinine and excess minerals!**

This ends processing **Procedure A**. You may stop here and cook your meat.

If you plan to fry your meat, be sure to place the drained meat on a small stack of paper towels, and blot off excess moisture before frying, to avoid spattering. Season as desired.

*NOTE - If you wish to lower the creatine content further, before it is eaten, proceed directly from **step** 4 to **Procedure B**.

Procedure B—
1. Placed the meat from **Step 4 (Procedure A)** into a minimum of 1 liter of water heated to between 170 - 180°F (light simmer - not boiling!).
2. Stir for approximately three to four minutes.
3. Drain into a clean colander or sieve.
4. Blot dry on a small stack of paper towels and serve.

Meat processed through **Procedure B** is cooked (if the meat was sliced into 1/8" thickness). If the slice thickness was 1/4" thick or greater, check the doneness of the meat by slicing several of the thicker pieced in half and observe the center for 'pinkness'. Be sure to cook any underdone chicken before eating.

Refrigerate any unused processed meat (from **Procedure A or B**) immediately. Use within 24 hours, or meat may be frozen for later use.

Recipe Tips for After Processing
1) After **Procedure A**, strips can be fried in low sodium, no trans fatty acids margarine, on low heat, just long enough to

give the chicken a good taste. Be sure to use your favorite seasonings as desired.

2) After **Procedure B**, pat strips dry, chill, then use in salad, or sandwiches. Strips can also be skewed, dipped in B.B.Q. sauce or a sauce of your choosing, then eaten.

Snappy Chicken Kabobs
Ingredients:
1 lb of sliced processed (Procedure A or B) chicken strips
cranberry sauce
white wine
lemon juice
pineapple slices
any color peppers cubed into 1 inch cubes

Combine the ingredients (cranberry sauce, white wine, lemon juice) in a small bowl. Thread the chicken, pineapple, and peppers on bamboo skewers. Season lightly with poultry seasoning and sage to taste. Place skewered meat slices in a baking dish. Glaze with a mixture of cranberry-orange relish, and cover with the wine/cranberry mixture. Cover dish with a vented cover and microwave on high until done (especially if the meat used is from Procedure A). Let stand covered for approximately 2 minutes after cooking before serving.

Cackling Good Rice Dish
Here is a dish that can be served any time
Ingredients:
1 lb of chicken strips (from Procedure A) spiced as follows:
> Poultry seasoning
> Sage
> Mrs. Dash (if desired)
> Black pepper (if desired)

Cook instant rice (according to instructions) until almost done. Then place in an oven/microwave safe dish and add one small can of mushroom soupe and chicken strips. Cook in the oven (at 325°F or 350°F) or in the microwave until meat is done.

PROCESSED MEATS

After processing, the meat will appear somewhat lighter in color. This is normal.

HAM (CURED)

Approximate creatine and mineral concentration per 100 grams (about 3 1/2 ounces) of cured ham, consumed as is, without special processing.

290 mg of Creatine
K – 292   P – 250   Na – 1104

Approximate creatine and mineral content remaining in 100 grams of thinly sliced (1/8" inch thickness) cured ham slices, after meat has been prepared according to the following procedure:

After Processing   Reduction Potential
58 mg of Creatine   80%
Minerals Remaining and Reduction Potential
K   P   Na   K   P   Na
174 mg 186 mg 320 mg   40%   26%   71%

Processing Instructions:
(Be sure to follow safe meat handling procedures at all times!)
NOTE - For easier slicing, this author recommends that the cured ham be lightly frozen before slicing.

1. Remove lightly frozen cured ham from its package and discard the package. Slice ham into 1/8" slices
2. Rinse under warm tap water (approximately 100°F), for 15 – 20 seconds.
3. Heat a minimum of 1 liter of water to between 170 - 180°F (lightly simmer - not boiling!).
4. Place up to 1 pound of rinsed ham slices in the lightly simmering water and stir for approximately two minutes.
5. Drain into a clean colander or sieve—**do not keep or use the water, it contains creatine/creatinine and excess minerals!**
6. Blot dry on a small stack of paper towels and serve.

NOTE - Cured ham processed longer than 6 minutes, in the above fashion, will be tasteless.

Be sure to refrigerate any uneaten meat. Cured ham that has been processed in the above manner is very perishable. Be sure to use within 24 hours or freeze any uneaten portion.

Recipe Tips for After Processing
Processed ham is very versatile. Processed ham can be used in:
1) Sandwiches – make toasted ham and cheese sandwiches. Be sure to use your favorite condiments.

2) Marinate until warm in no trans fatty acids margarine. Serve with scrambled eggs and toast, if desired.
3) Add ham to sliced potatoes and milk (with processed cheese, if desired) to make a scalloped potato. Use your favorite recipe to add "zip" to the final taste if desired.
4) Add to cooked vegetables for a light flavor.
5) Add processed ham to sauerkraut while cooking.
6) Use in all your favorite recipes that call for ham, either slices or cubes.

Be creative! The uses for processed ham are only limited by your imagination.

WIENERS (PORK)

Approximate creatine and mineral concentration per 100 grams (about 3 1/2 ounces) of boiled wieners, without special processing.

91 mg of Creatine
K – 155 mg   P – 222 mg   Na - 1379

Approximate creatine and mineral content remaining in 100 grams of thinly sliced (cross-cut - 1/8" inch thickness) wieners, after meat has been prepared according to the following procedure:

After Processing   Reduction Potential
46 mg of Creatine   49%

Minerals Remaining and Reduction Potential
K	P	Na	K	P	Na
88 mg	187 mg	840 mg	43%	16%	39%

Processing Instructions:
(Be sure to follow safe meat handling procedures at all times!)
NOTE - For easier slicing, this author recommends that the wieners be lightly frozen before slicing. For ease of slicing, this author recommends cutting crosswise.

1. Remove lightly frozen wieners from their package and discard the package. Slice into 1/8" slices.
2. Rinse under warm tap water (approximately 100°F), for 15 – 20 seconds.
3. Heat a minimum of 1 liter of water to between 170 - 180°F (lightly simmer - not boiling!).
4. Place up to 1 pound of rinsed, sliced wieners in the lightly simmering water and stir for approximately 5 minutes.
5. Drain into a clean colander or sieve—**do not keep or use the water, it contains creatine/creatinine and excess minerals!**
6. Blot dry on a small stack of paper towels and serve.

NOTE - The Wiener's taste **does not** diminish substantially even after processing as long as 7 minutes.

Be sure to refrigerate any uneaten meat. Wieners that have been processed in the above manner are very perishable. Be sure to use 24 hours or freeze any uneaten portion.

Recipe Tips for After Processing
Processed wieners make:

1) Sandwiches – use as they are or place in a food processor (a hand grinder can also be used) and blend into a fine paste with Lite Miracle Whip dressing, minced onion, and dry mustard,
2) Alternately, they are good served with scrambled eggs,
3) They season sauerkraut,
4) Cubed processed wieners can be used in salads, and even served as appetizers on crackers or with (Processed) cheese,

5) They make a great tasting macaroni dish with mayonnaise, peas, carrots and chunks of (Processed cheese) on top,
6) Mixed in to any rice (wild or domestic) dish,
7) Blends well with other ingredients in Taco or on any meat Pizza,
8) Can be covered with a tomato-paste glaze and eaten with spaghetti,

And many many more uses…just use your imagination with this one!

CHEESE

Cheese sheets will loose their shape during processing. It is normal to see a milky substance (whey) cloud the bowl during processing.

Processed cheese makes great tub cheese and can be used for a variety of dishes. Cheese can be soft frozen, cubed, and stored frozen for later use in a number of dishes.

CHEESE
(American Processed Cheese - slices)

Approximate creatine and mineral concentration per 100 grams (about 3 1/2 ounces or about 5 sheets of American Processed Cheese) without special processing.
    26 mg of Creatine
K – 247 mg   P – 471 mg   Na – 1054 mg

Approximate creatine and mineral content remaining in 100 grams (about 5 sheets) of American Processed Cheese after processing according to the following procedure:

After Processing   **Reduction Potential**
16 mg of Creatine   38%
Minerals Remaining and Reduction Potential

K	P	Na	K	P	Na
54 mg	352 mg	484 mg	78%	25%	54%

Processing Instructions:
1. Remove American Processed Cheese slices from their wrappers and discard the wrapper.
2. Place up to 1 pound of slices in a minimum of 2 liters of warm tap water (approximately 100°F), stir **carefully**, then allow cheese to settle and stand for 1 hour on the counter.

NOTE - Cheese slices will settle and stick to the sides and bottom of the container—this is normal. Cheese will quickly become gummy. Do not try to move the cheese during the processing procedure.

3. Drain by slowly powering the water away, taking care not to let any lose cheese slices slip from the container.
4. When the last visible water has drained away, using a kitchen spatula or meat turner, slide the cheese from the container onto several thickness of paper toweling.
5. Allow the cheese to stand for several minutes. If the cheese was unusually wet when it was removed, pace a layer of paper toweling on top of the cheese and blot gently.
6. After most of the moisture has been removed, scoop cheese into a container and store in the refrigerator.

NOTE - Cheese thus processes makes great 'tub cheese' with a very mild taste.

The cheese can now be mixed with mayonnaise to make a spread, melted to make a dip, or added to other foods. Be sure to keep any uneaten cheese refrigerated. Cheese that has been processed in the above manner is very perishable and will sour. This author has never attempted to keep cheese in the refrigerator, after it has been processed, longer than 3 days. Cheese that has been processed can be frozen and used later.

Recipe Tips for After Processing
This processed cheese can be used, as is, for bread spread. It is also very good mixed with pimientos, minced onion, sugar, and Lite Miracle Whip and spread on crackers or bread.

Spread Ingredients:
1 lb of (processed) cheese
1 small jar of pimientos
1 or 2 tbs of minced onion
1 tsp (or to taste), sugar

Add enough Lite Miracle Whip salad dressing to make it spreadable. Mix until well blended. This cheese can be used in all of your favorite recipes.

Melted Cheese Dip
Any amount of cheese may be melted to make a dip. A cheese dip may be spiced up by adding any one of the following:
garlic powder
fresh ground pepper
chopped green onions
milk
pimientos

several drops of lemon juice
various herbs

Uses for melted (processed) cheese are endless, and limited only by your imagination.

MY PERSONAL DIETARY INSTRUCTIONS

Meat(s) I usually eat:
1.

2.

3.

4.

5.

6.

7.

MY DIETITIAN'S RECOMMENDATIONS

A. _____

B. _____

C. _____

D. _____

E. _____

F. _____

G. _____

ADDITIONAL NOTES

Conclusions

Consuming a total dietary selection of creatine reduced meats is expected to have a positive impact on the renal patients nutritional profile, as well as their problematic serum creatinine values

About the Author

Wendy Lou Jones was born in 1956 in St. Cloud Minnesota. She began her Bachelors study in biological science at Southwest State University in 1974, Masters studies at South Dakota State University in 1979, and Ph.D. studies in Calgary Canada in 1982.

A dynamic, success oriented clinical and research investigator in the fields of renal research and biotechnology, Wendy Jones has held positions in the US, Canada, and Austria, amassing more than 20 years of combined laboratory experience in Alberta Canada in oncology, at Minnesota's Mayo Clinic in arthritis and transgenic research, as medical/technical writer in one of Vienna Austria's largest pharmaceuticals, as Royal Knight's clinical trials manager, as scientific manuscript reviewer for the National Science Foundation, and as editor of the e-Business quarterly.

Wendy Jones is currently the president and CEO of the Royal Knight, Inc., a company whose primary interest is in promoting renal research in the field of kidney cell and tissue regeneration. Wendy Jones actively writes clinical protocols, supervises clinical studies, and provides direction and assistance to other companies seeking those expertise

REFERENCES

Acchiardo SR, Moore LW, Latour PA: Malnutrition as the main factor in morbidity, and mortality of hemodialysis patients. Kidney Int 1983; 24:S199-S203, (suppl 16)

Ahmed KJ, Kopple JD: Nutrition in Maintenance Hemodialysis Patients. Factors Altering Nutrient Requirements in Maintenance Hemodialysis Patients, in Kopple JD, Massry SG (eds.): Nutritional Management of Renal Disease. Williams and Wilkins, Baltimore, Maryland, 1997, pp. 563-600

Anonymous: Hemodialysis Outbreak. MMWR 1998; 47(23):483-484, (editorial)

Anonymous. Understanding Food Labels. ADA (food label pamphlet) 1998.

Balsom PD, Söderlund K, Ekblom B. Creatine in humans with special reference to creatine supplementation. Sports Med.1994; 18(4):268-280

Delanghe J, De Slypere J-P, De Buyzere M, et al. Normal reference values for creatine, creatinine, and carnitine are lower in vegetarians. Clin Chem 1989; 35:1802-1803

Felton JS, Fultz E, Dolbeare FA, Knize MG. Effect of microwave pretreatment on heterocyclic aromatic amine mutagens/carcinogens in fried beef patties. Fd Chem Toxic 1994; 32(10): 897-903

Hoogwerf BJ, Laine DC, Greene E. Urine C-peptide and creatinine (Jaffe method) excretion in healthy young adults on varied diets: sustained effects of varied carbohydrate, protein and meat content. Am J Clin Nutr 1986; 43:350-360

Jacobsen FK, Christensen CK, Morgensen CE, Andreasen F, Heilskov NSC. Postprandial serum creatinine increase in normal subjects after eating cooked meat. Proc EDTA 1979; 16:506-512

Jägerstad M, Skog K. Formation of Meat Mutagens, in Friedman M. (ed): Nutritional and Toxicological Consequences of Food Processing. Plenum Oress, New York, 1991, pp. 83-105

Jones WL, Demineralization of a Wide Variety of Foods for the Renal Patient. J Renal Nutr 2001; 11(2):90-96

> (a) Disease Outcome Quality Initiative (DOQI). Management of Protein and Energy Intake. Dietary

Protein Intake (DPI) in Maintenance Hemodialysis (MHD). AJKD 2000; 35(No.6 − suppl. 2):S40-41.

(b) Kidney Disease Outcome Quality Initiative (DOQI). Management of Protein and Energy Intake. Dietary Protein Intake (DPI) for Chronic Peritoneal Dialysis (CPD). AJKD 2000; 35(No.6 − suppl. 2):S42-43.

Levey S. Perrone R. Madias N. Serum creatinine and function. Annu Rev Med 1988; 39:465-490

Maiorca R, Brunori G, Zubani R, et al: Predictive value of dialysis adequacy and nutritional indices for mortality and morbidity in CAPD and HD patients. A longitudinal study. Nephrol Dial Transplant 1995; 10:2295-2305

Mayersohn M, Conrad KA, Achari R. The influence of a cooked meat meal on creatinine plasma concentration and creatinine clearance. Brit J Clin Pharm 1983; 15(2):227-230

Vikse R, Joner PE. Mutagenicity, Creatine and nutrient content of pan-fried meat from various animal species. Acta Vet Scand 1993; 24(4):363-370

Printed in the United Kingdom
by Lightning Source UK Ltd.
104388UKS00002B/48